I H♥TE RUNNING

AND
YOU CAN TOO

I H♥TE RUNNING

AND
YOU CAN TOO

*How to Get Started, Keep Going, and
Make Sense of an Irrational Passion*

BRENDAN LEONARD

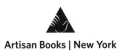

Artisan Books | New York

Library of Congress Cataloging-in-Publication Data

Names: Leonard, Brendan, author.
Title: I Hate Running and You Can Too : How to Get Started, Keep Going, and Make Sense of an Irrational Passion / Brendan Leonard.
Description: New York, NY : Artisan, a division of Workman Publishing Co.,Inc., 2021.
Identifiers: LCCN 2020042966 | ISBN 9781579659882 (paperback)
Subjects: LCSH: Long-distance running. | Running--Psychological aspects. | Runners (Sports)
Classification: LCC GV1062 .L46 2021 | DDC 796.4201/9--dc23
LC record available at https://lccn.loc.gov/2020042966

Design by Jane Treuhaft

Artisan books are available at special discounts when purchased in bulk for premiums and sales promotions as well as for fund-raising or educational use. Special editions or book excerpts also can be created to specification. For details, contact the Special Sales Director at the address below, or send an e-mail to specialmarkets@workman.com.

For speaking engagements, contact speakersbureau@workman.com.

Published by Artisan
A division of Workman Publishing Co., Inc.
225 Varick Street
New York, NY 10014-4381
artisanbooks.com

Artisan is a registered trademark of Workman Publishing Co., Inc.
Published simultaneously in Canada by Thomas Allen & Son, Limited

Printed in China
First printing, February 2021

10 9 8 7 6 5 4 3 2

TO ANYONE WHO WONDERS IF
THEY CAN GO A LITTLE FARTHER

CONTENTS

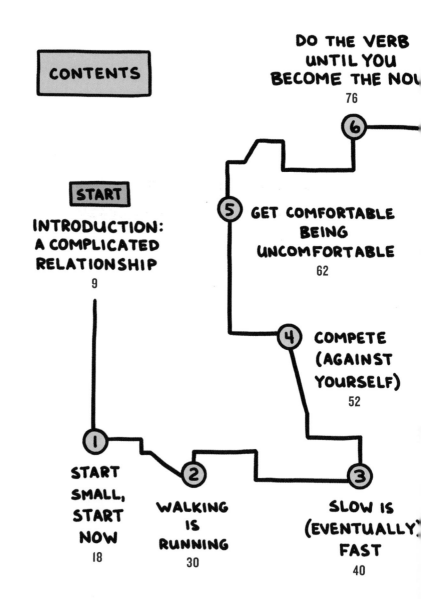

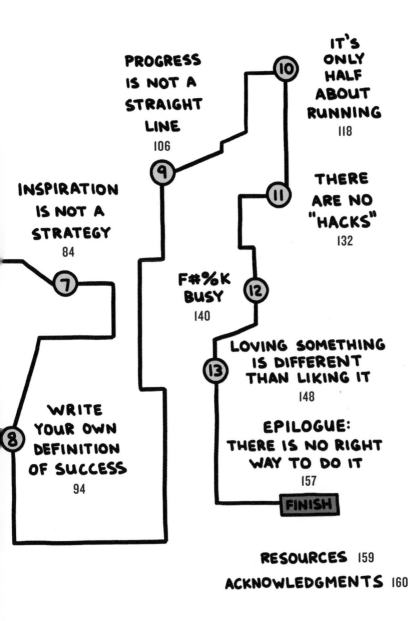

INTRODUCTION

A COMPLICATED RELATIONSHIP

I hate running. Frequently, actually. Usually three or four times a week.

I don't hate running the entire time—there are moments where I actually sort of enjoy it. When I'm finished, I like having run. I just don't like doing it compared to doing other things, like eating pizza or taking naps, which are a lot more fun and a lot less effort.

I hate running dozens of miles every week and thousands of miles per year. I have hated it for 3 miles after work on a Tuesday around the park near my house, I've hated it for 26.2 miles through New York City, I've hated it for 100 miles straight in the mountains of North Carolina, and I've hated it in Wyoming and Colorado on other occasions.

I'm not a professional runner or even a consistent lifelong runner—I sort of rediscovered running in my midthirties through a curiosity about ultrarunning. I'd spent hundreds of days in the mountains doing almost every other sport in my career as an adventure writer—mountaineering, backcountry skiing, rock climbing, backpacking, cycling, hiking, bikepacking, and white-water rafting—but I'd only done a little bit of trail running. I'd known about people who ran races longer than marathons—31 miles, 50 miles, even 100 miles and longer—and I'd always wondered if I could too.

On my high school track team, I proved to be ineffective at running distances longer than 200 meters. After a few 400-meter-dash performances during which I believed it might be possible to actually vomit a lung, I told my coach, "Four hundred meters is long distance," and he limited me to races 200 meters and under. I mostly gave up running after high school, choosing to instead take up smoking one pack of cigarettes every day for six years, which turned out to be a terrible idea. At twenty-six years old, I knew I had to quit smoking, so I signed up for a marathon, thinking training for a 26.2-mile race would finally inspire me to quit. It did. I finished the marathon and rewarded myself with a nine-year break from any sort of regular running. I stayed active doing everything else in the outdoors, including the occasional trail run, and finally scratched that "could I finish an ultramarathon?" itch in 2015, by signing up for a 50-kilometer race. At mile 26, I almost quit because of an excruciating pain in my left knee, but was able to walk, massage my IT band, jog, and then finally run to the finish line. Within two years of that race, I was lining up for a 100-miler (which I finished—but barely).

Since then, I've run dozens of ultramarathons and marathons and run thousands of miles. I've spent time exploring the diversity of running, from the short weekday runs I do by myself to the New York City Marathon with 53,000 other people, to 100-mile sufferfests on mountain trails. I approach it like I do everything that requires effort and commitment, and I speak about the parallels between work and running to audiences whenever I can. I assure these people that if they hate running, that's okay—I do too.

You might ask: Why do I do something I hate so much, so often? That's a perfectly valid question. I guess as an adult I realized I had to do some sort of regular exercise for health and sanity, and running seemed to be the best option. Yes, I hate it most of the time, but maybe once during every run, I have a few seconds, or a minute or two, where I find myself thinking, "You know, this isn't so bad."

Some might say I'm a bit of a masochist. If I sat next to someone on an airplane and happened to tell them how much I run, and that person said, "Wow, that sounds like a dumb hobby," I would respect their opinion because I share that exact opinion the majority of the time.

In all the races I've run, though, I've noticed something: A lot of people run. Are they, like me, simply masochists?

Probably a little bit, but that's not it. We all run at different speeds and we're different shapes and different sizes, but we all have the same itch, and we all scratch that itch with running. I'm certainly not going to speak for every other runner, but I will say that knowing there are others with this same irrational passion for running long distances makes me feel less alone while doing this thing that I hate but kind of like.

Since the running boom of the 1970s and '80s, running has remained one of the most popular forms of exercise in the world—this is according to FitBit data we now have access to, not just people saying "Running? Sure, I run." So why do we run? Well, running is cheaper than buying home gym equipment, for one thing. And getting set up is a lot less complicated. You don't need anything other than a pair of running shoes (and some people would argue you don't even need them), and you can run almost anywhere. You can run as long or as short as you want, as fast or as slow as you want, by yourself or with friends, at five a.m. or midnight. Running gives you time alone with your thoughts and gives you the freedom to have one thing in your life that you do just for you. And you can start running when you're six years old or sixty-five.

The other thing I have noticed about those of us with a passion for running: When you show up at a marathon, or a 10K or 5K, most of the other people there—like me—are

To call running "fun" would be a misuse of the word. Running can be "enjoyable." Running can be "rejuvenating." But in a pure sense of the word, running is not fun.

—DEAN KARNAZES, *Ultramarathon Man: Confessions of an All-Night Runner*

not in danger of qualifying for the Olympics any time soon. Sure, a few dozen or a couple hundred people at the front of the pack in any race are uniquely fast athletes, but the rest of us are regular folks who have jobs and families and mortgages, and we all have this weird hobby of running as far as we can. We train for weeks or months to attempt a distance that many people (including ourselves) might think is irrational for anyone who is not getting chased by bears or lions or other megafauna.

I suspect most of us runners have a complicated relationship with running—you could call it a love-hate relationship, but I think it's more nuanced than that. If running were a person I was dating, I would definitely have broken up with that person long ago. But running is more like a weird friend I keep hanging out with and who is good for me in a really strange way—despite being pretty unlikable most of the time. In 2017, I started spelling out this love-hate relationship as I H♥TE RUNNING, so I could put it on a T-shirt and communicate my feelings in the most direct and accurate way possible.

Everybody should try running. And when I say try it, I mean do it long enough that you get through the part where it sucks and into the fleeting but noticeable part where you actually think it's fun. Because during every run, for a few seconds or a few minutes, you have a moment where it feels really good. You forget about the discomfort and you find rhythm, maybe some grace, and a feeling of strength and confidence as you move as well as you'll ever move doing anything. And that's one of the best reasons to run.

AN IRRATIONAL PASSION INVOLVES IRRATIONAL DISTANCES

Let's be real here: If you're not late for a bus or a flight, running more than a few hundred feet is pretty irrational. We have dozens of highly efficient ways to travel, and if you're traveling by foot, walking is usually more than sufficient to get the job done.

I have run all the irrational distances from 1 mile up to 102.9 miles, and what I discovered is this: Once you run a distance, it ceases to become irrational. It seems ridiculously far before you do it and maybe even while you're

IF YOU ARE A PERSON WHO CAN CURRENTLY RUN	IT SEEMS REASONABLY POSSIBLE TO BECOME A PERSON WHO CAN RUN	BUT ONLY A COMPLETE PSYCHOPATH WOULD BE ABLE TO RUN
0 MILES	1 MILE	3 MILES
1 MILE	3 MILES	6 MILES
3 MILES	6 MILES	13.1 MILES
6 MILES	13.1 MILES	26.2 MILES
13.1 MILES	26.2 MILES	31 MILES
26.2 MILES	31 MILES	50 MILES
31 MILES	50 MILES	62 MILES
50 MILES	62 MILES	100 MILES
62 MILES	100 MILES	>100 MILES
100 MILES	> 100 MILES	?

doing it, but the next day or two days later, you find yourself thinking, "That wasn't so bad." And maybe you start thinking about the next distance you can run.

For the purposes of this book, "long distance" is not an objective term. If you don't currently have a regular running habit, "long distance" refers to anything farther than however far you would run to catch a plane or a bus. If you've run a 5K recently, "long distance" refers to anything farther than that. If you've run a half-marathon, it refers to any distance farther than 13.1 miles. And so on. When you read this book and you see the phrase "long distance," think of whatever distance seems like a challenge to you.

WHAT IS AND *IS NOT* IN THIS BOOK

This is not a how-to book or a memoir of a very fast person who has stood on podiums at the finish lines of races. It will not tell you how to train for a race, how to eat during, before, or after running and/or racing, or what kind of shoes to buy or clothes to wear, or what kind of stretches to do before or after running.

This book is intended to convince you that you *can* run an irrational distance, whatever that distance is. And if you're already convinced, this book will help you explain to yourself, or to other people, why you have such an irrational passion for running. I also hope you'll find some motivation, some levity, maybe a handful of laughs, and moments of recognition in these pages.

I hope to convince you to h♥te running too.

If you find yourself hating running and quitting early, just keep at it. Running takes time to become enjoyable. It's not a surgical strike; it's a war of attrition.

—MATTHEW INMAN (aka The Oatmeal)

I. START

SMALL, START NOW

Start small, start now. This is much better than, "start big, start later." One advantage is that you don't have to start perfect. You can merely start.

—SETH GODIN

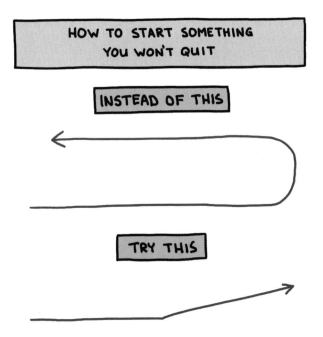

HOW TO START SOMETHING YOU WON'T QUIT

INSTEAD OF THIS

TRY THIS

Alex Honnold is famous for climbing the sheer face of Yosemite's 3,000-foot El Capitan without a rope. He is significantly less famous for gently, perhaps even unintentionally, nudging his mother, Dierdre Wolownick, from running zero miles per week at age fifty-five to becoming a marathon runner. In her memoir, *The Sharp End of Life*, Wolownick recalls her evening walk spontaneously turning into a mile-long run with the family dog. She arrived home to tell her son about it. He shrugged and said, "Cool. If you can do one, you can do one and a half." A few nights later, after she reported to Alex that she and the dog had just run a mile and a half, he responded: "Cool. If you can do a mile and a half, you can do two."

After progressing to 2 miles, then 3, she ran her first 10K in jeans and a flannel shirt. Just over a year later, after training for twenty weeks, she ran her first marathon. Wolownick, with no intention to run really long distances in her fifties, started small and eventually went big.

More than half a million people in the United States finish a marathon each year. Almost none of those people do it without running a bunch of miles in the months beforehand. At some point, every person was running zero miles per week. And then they ran one mile a few times, and eventually decided they could run a mile and a half. And so on. A long race, whether your definition of "long" is 6.2 miles or 100 miles, starts with running (or walking) a much shorter distance, one time. And then doing it again. And again. You do a small thing once, twice, three times, and you start stacking those small things on top of one another, or depositing them in a metaphorical account, and they start to add up.

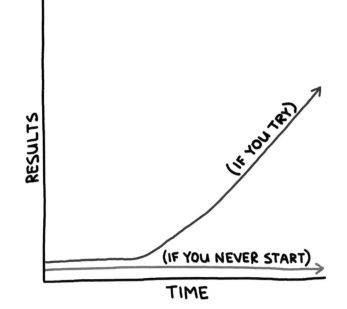

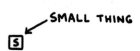
SMALL THING

TWO SMALL THINGS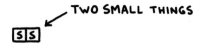

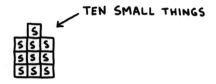
TEN SMALL THINGS

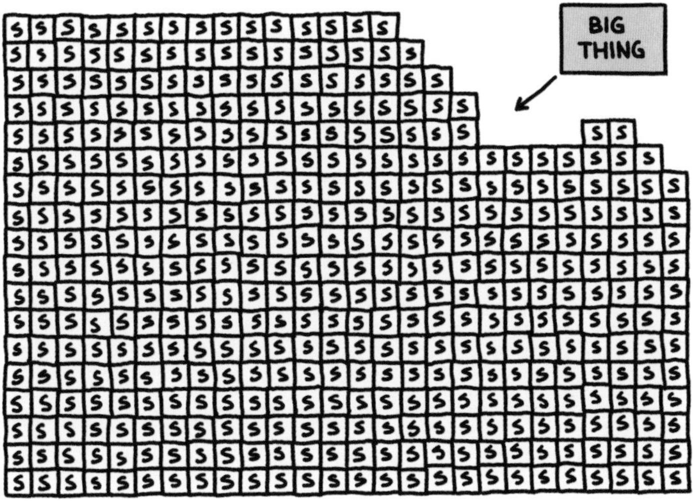
BIG THING

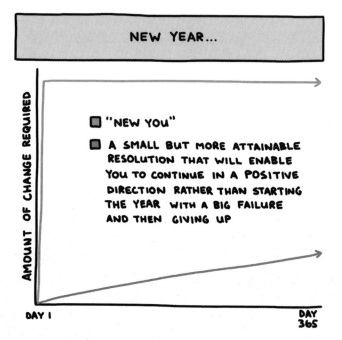

Human beings generally suck at keeping New Year's resolutions because we often make them too big and too abrupt, and after a week or so, we hit a bump in the road, get discouraged, and abandon our big new change altogether. We find that our extreme new diet is hard to stick with, or our new exercise routine increases our time at the gym 1,000 percent over the previous year, or that as it turns out, eating raw kale three times a day, seven days a week, just isn't bringing us happiness after all. "New year, new you" is a ridiculous, almost always unattainable concept (unless you're in the FBI's Witness Protection Program, in which case you have reason to be way more optimistic about the idea of a 100 percent "new you"). "New year, gradually improving you" is way more realistic—and it allows you to slowly grow into something and keep going, as opposed to taking on a difficult, complete transformation, and giving up after a few weeks.

So wherever you're starting on your progression to running some irrational distance, whether it's 6 miles or 26.2 miles, start with something rational. As Leo Babauta, creator of the *Zen Habits* blog, puts it, "Make it so easy you can't say no."

2. WA

KING IS RUNNING

I've been on the U.S. Olympic Team and have run for more than 50 years, and I didn't know that there was a running rule book that excludes walking.

—JEFF GALLOWAY, when someone says, "If you take walk breaks, you're not a real runner," *The Run-Walk-Run Method*

I n preparing to run my first marathon in 2006, I made a promise to myself: No matter what, I would run every step of the race. It didn't have to be fast, but I wanted to get to the finish line knowing I had actually "run a marathon."

And I stuck with it. Until mile 5, when I tried to jog through a water station, grab a 6-ounce cup of water, and drink it without breaking my stride. About half of the water spilled onto my face and down my shirt. I amended my strategy: I would run every step of the race, except when drinking cups of water and/or sports drinks, which were served every 5 miles.

From then on, I ran every step of the race, except for the 100 feet or so when I was grabbing a cup of water from an aid station. This strategy worked a lot better than my original plan, as I was able to actually consume fluids instead of dumping them onto my shirt, where they could not be absorbed into my body.

About 3 miles from the end of the course, when everyone in the race had spread out and I was running mostly alone and wondering if the finish line would ever appear, a runner passed me. About 150 feet ahead of me, she stopped jogging and slowed to a walk. I caught up to her and passed her. A few hundred feet later, she passed me again, and a while later, slowed to a walk again. We continued this pattern for a while. She was walking and running, and I was still determined to run the whole thing.

Who was right? Both of us. More than a decade later, I can't remember if she finished ahead of me, or if I finished ahead of her. How much either of us walked or ran didn't matter then, and it doesn't matter now.

I didn't know it at the time, but walking is a big part of a lot of people's marathon strategies. They run three minutes, then walk one minute, then repeat. Or they run four minutes, then walk one minute, then repeat. Or they run one minute, walk the next minute, and continue until they're done with the race, or some other version of this strategy, which was popularized by Jeff Galloway, Olympian, coach, and author, and has since been used by thousands of runners.

Here's what a half-marathon looks like running the whole distance nonstop at ten-minute miles versus breaking it up into chunks of running for nine minutes at a time, followed by a two-minute walk break, then repeating that sequence for the entire race (except for the final 1.1 miles):

13.1 MILES @ 10:00 PER MILE:

= 2:11:00 HALF-MARATHON TIME

13.1 MILES @:
■ RUNNING @ 10:00 PER MILE
□ WALKING @ 20:00 PER MILE

= 2:24:06 HALF-MARATHON TIME

Those walk breaks, at a twenty-minute-per-mile pace, add some time, but not that much, right? A 2:24:06 finish time is very respectable.

Here's what the same distance looks like if you go out hard and run nine-minute miles for the first 10 miles of the race, then blow up and walk the final 3.1 miles.

13.1 MILES @:
■ RUNNING @ 9:00 PER MILE
□ WALKING @ 20:00 PER MILE

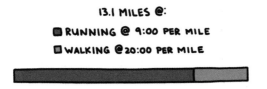

= 2:32:00 HALF-MARATHON TIME

It's easy to assume that anyone who completes a race runs the entire thing. But that would be wrong. Sure, Shalane Flanagan ran *all* of the New York City Marathon when she won it in 2017, as did Eliud Kipchoge when he broke the marathon world record in 2018. But most of us should give ourselves some slack. As Jeff Galloway has said, there is no rule book for running that excludes walking.

If you explore ultramarathons, you'll discover how much walking ultrarunners do—even elite runners in mountainous 100-mile races. The terrain, the long hours, and the calorie consumption required to finish necessitate walking. In order to keep moving and actually finish (instead of blowing up partway through), a common strategy is to walk the uphills and run the flats and downhills. I think of the three pillars of ultrarunning like this:

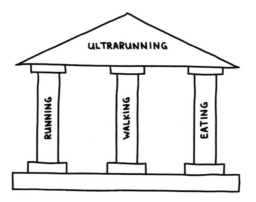

If I had never ever run an ultramarathon, I might have assumed all running looked like this:

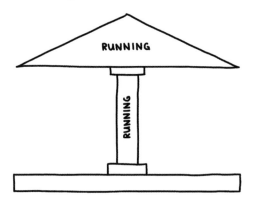

Of course, for a short jog around the park near my house, that's sustainable. But when I get into longer distances, a single-pillar approach is much less stable. So my running usually looks more like this:

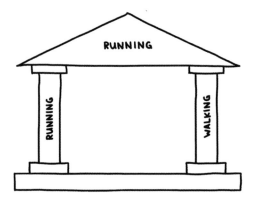

Here's something to think about: The men's world record holder in the 50-kilometer (about 31.25 miles) racewalk, Yohann Diniz, would qualify for the Boston Marathon if you use his 50K walking time (3 hours, 32 minutes, 33 seconds) to calculate his marathon running time (2 hours, 59 minutes, 39 seconds); on the women's side of racewalking, the top seven women's 50K racewalk times would qualify for Boston, which is sort of mind-bending. That's a lot of math to say: There are a handful of people who could get into the Boston Marathon, one of the most prestigious running events in the world, by walking every step of a marathon.

World-record racewalking aside, if you're not currently running regularly, walking regularly is a good way to get started. It gets your body used to spending time on your feet (especially if you work many hours sitting at a desk), and walking a mile or two a few times a week can get you used to building exercise time into your schedule. When you decide to transition from regular walks three or four times a week to regular runs three or four times a week, the changeover will be easier and you'll probably enjoy getting through the miles more quickly.

Allowing yourself to walk makes running less daunting, less restrictive, less all-or-nothing. There are no rules, and no one's keeping track but you, so figure out what works and use it to log some miles.

A decade after I finished that first marathon and discovered the joy of walking, I started running ultramarathons. When it comes up in conversation that I have done a 50-mile race or a 100-mile race, and someone says, "Fifty miles? I could never run that far." I always reply, "I can't either. Almost nobody does. We walk. Some of us walk a lot."

Speed isn't nearly as important as not stopping.

You can eat while you're walking. You can cry while you're walking. I am proof that you can puke and walk at the same time. There's no reason to stop.

—MEGHAN HICKS, editor of IRunFar.com; finisher of dozens of ultramarathons

3. SLOW IS (B

ENTUALLY) FAST

Run slow to run fast.

—Old running adage

I f you ever hire a guide to help you climb a big snowy mountain taller than 14,000 feet, like Mt. Rainier or Mt. Shasta, the guide will almost always do one very valuable thing for you: Set the cruise control. Over the past century, mountain guides discovered something when taking groups of clients up big mountains—that going slow and keeping rest breaks to a minimum was way more efficient than going hard and having to stop often.

The "guide pace" can seem slow to a client, especially down low on the mountain, but at 11,000 or 12,000 feet, after everyone's been climbing what feels like snowy stairs for hours upon hours, the strategy proves itself. In the thinner air, instead of taking ten steps, then stopping for ten seconds to catch your breath, you're plodding steadily upward, slowly but gradually, and keeping your momentum going.

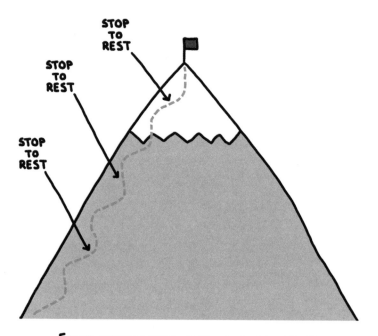

[THE PRAGMATIC AND SUSTAINABLE
PACE SET BY THE MOUNTAIN GUIDE]

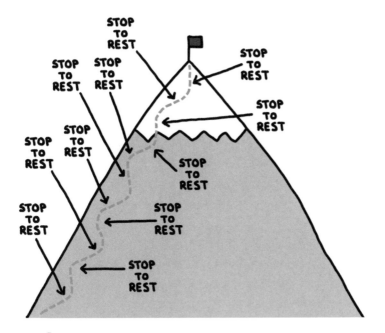

[THE ASPIRATIONAL AND UNSUSTAINABLE
PACE SET BY THE UNGUIDED CLIENT]

If you've ever driven a long distance in a car full of family members, you probably know why this strategy works: Fewer stops mean fewer chances for extended delays, because no stop is ever very quick. If you pull over to stop so Kid #1 can use the restroom, everyone gets out of the car. Then Kid #2 wants a Slurpee and you spend ten minutes negotiating, and pretty soon you've stopped for thirty minutes. And if you stop more than once, the delays just build, build, and build.

What does this have to do with distance running? It just means that you don't need to worry so much about going fast—not stopping is the key. Plenty of experts would tell you that running fast all the time leads to burnout and is not a good strategy to get faster. I'm not necessarily an expert on training strategies, but I'd also ask, what's the rush? My run—once I finally drag my ass out the door to do it—is often the best part of my day. Why make it a painful thirty-minute run when I can make it a (slightly less painful) thirty-five-minute run? More important, I'm way more likely to finish an easy run than a hard run. I have, more than once, taken off fast on a 7-mile run, and, once I'm huffing and puffing, I let the voice in my head talk me down to 6 miles . . . and then, maybe 5 miles sounds good enough . . . actually, 4 miles. This type of thing, in our mountain-climbing analogy, looks like this:

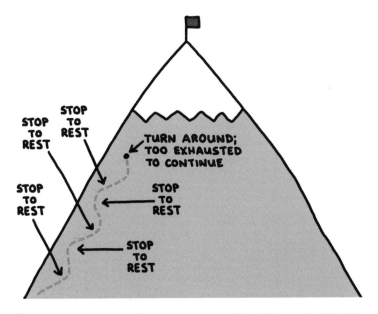

[THE PREMATURE ENDING THAT OFTEN RESULTS FROM SETTING AN UNSUSTAINABLE PACE]

Running coach David Roche, coauthor of *The Happy Runner*, who works with elite runners and regular folks alike, recommends that a minimum of 80 percent of your running should be easy (that is, you should be able to have a conversation while running), no matter what training approach you use.

Now, there's nothing wrong with wanting to run fast, whether you want to qualify for the Boston Marathon or knock a few seconds off your turkey trot time from last year. But becoming fast isn't the only way to enjoy running. And oftentimes, as more than a few champion runners will tell you, forgetting about getting faster can, paradoxically, lead to getting faster.

Running responds to a sense of ease and smoothness. It seems like it's about pushing hard, but it's not. It's about changing what your "easy" is. It's about making running the same effort—or the same pace or the same output—take less energy.

—DAVID ROCHE

There's a common psychological concept called "the hedonic treadmill." An internet search will turn up dozens of articles about it, but the gist is this: The things we think will make us happy will only lead to a small, short-term bump in happiness before we return back to our normal level of happiness. The hedonic treadmill is often used to explain why more money (or more material things like nice cars, TVs, etc.) doesn't actually make us happy.

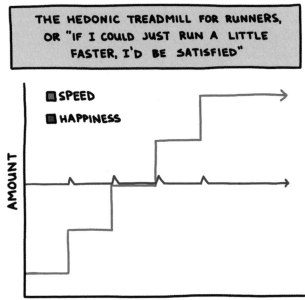

In Christopher McDougall's bestselling book *Born to Run*, the author meets with Micah True, aka Caballo Blanco, an American who followed Tarahumara runners to their home in Mexico's Copper Canyons to learn how they run long distances fast and joyfully. In relaying what he's learned, Caballo Blanco gives the author a mantra: "Easy, light, smooth, and fast." These are the four things a runner should try to achieve, in that order.

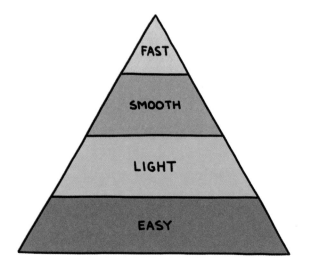

Easy is the base of that pyramid, because in Caballo Blanco's words, "You start with easy, because if that's all you get, that's not so bad." You can do easy runs until you're ready to build on that base of the pyramid, or you can simply enjoy easy running.

So maybe your hedonic treadmill chart looks more like this:

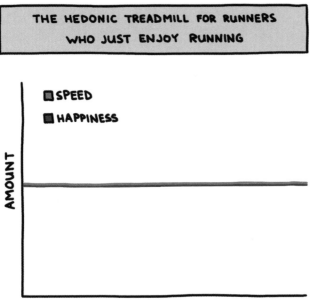

THE HEDONIC TREADMILL FOR RUNNERS
WHO JUST ENJOY RUNNING

■ SPEED
■ HAPPINESS

AMOUNT

TIME

If you learn to enjoy running, you'll want to keep doing it longer, and eventually you'll get better at it. Maybe you'll even become faster (whether you're trying to or not).

4. COMPETE (A

AINST YOURSELF)

*I'm not in competition with anybody.
I do my own thing.*

—BERNIE MAC

Just before the start of a race, whether it's a 5K, a marathon, or an ultramarathon, it's easy to catch yourself doing something really unhealthy and unproductive: looking around at all the other runners, checking them out, and wondering if they're fitter or faster than you or if they "deserve" to be there more than you do. Sure, many of them are faster than you. But none of them deserves to be there any more or any less than you do. I mean, sure, there are people at the front of the pack who will finish in half the time the rest of us do, and they'll win potentially thousands of dollars in prize money, so I guess you could say they're more professionally qualified to be there—but think about it this way: Everyone in that starting corral, whether they run five-minute miles or fourteen-minute miles, is hoping they won't have to stop to poop in the middle of the race. In that, we are all equal.

More than 50,000 people run the New York City Marathon each year. If you're lucky enough to be one of them, I'll bet you a dollar that you won't ever find yourself telling your grandkids, "I got 33,789th place that year, but if a couple things had gone a little differently for me, I could have gotten 32,372nd place." You're more likely to tell them about what a challenging, fun, and exciting experience it was. And when you go back to work the week after the race, your coworkers are not going ask you, "Did you win?"

Yes, it's called a "race," but who are you really competing with? Some people would say you're competing with the distance or the race course, and those things may both be true, but I'd say you're competing with slightly lesser versions of yourself. Picture something like what you see opposite.

Even if you never run a race, you might find yourself comparing yourself to other runners: those slightly more athletic-looking people in the park who run faster or who spent more money on running shorts. Again, don't do that. Of all the millions of people who go for a run every day, an overwhelming majority of us don't feel that we look very good when we run: We think we have a little bit too much jiggle, or we think we sweat too much, or we think we run too slowly, or we think we look a little funny when compared to that gazelle-like person we see once or twice a week on our running route. Okay, so we don't look so much like Olympic athletes. Most of us don't think we have what we imagine to be a "runner's body."

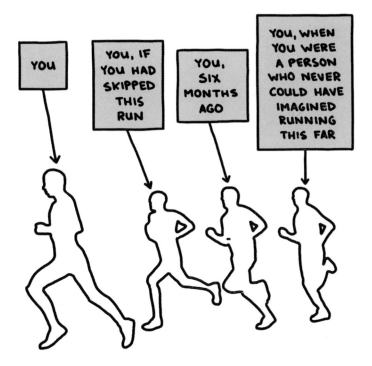

Here's a good saying to remind yourself: Any body that runs is a runner's body. If you run enough days per year, you'll see all shapes and sizes of people out running too, wearing all kinds of clothing, from top-of-the-line running gear to old cotton T-shirts and basketball shorts. We're all runners and we're all trying to improve just a little bit on the person we were yesterday, or last month, or last year.

Look, nobody ever says a grizzly bear has a "runner's body"—but in a footrace, a grizzly bear would absolutely kick the shit out of the fastest human ever. And the grizzly bear spends literally zero time training.

GRIZZLY BEAR	USAIN BOLT
7 FEET TALL 400-750 POUNDS 35 MPH	6 FEET, 5 INCHES TALL 207 POUNDS 27 MPH

If someday you run a race, you might be surprised at how many people line the streets to cheer for you and all the other runners. They don't care what place you're in, or how fast you're going. They're not cheering for you because you're winning the race; they're cheering for you because you had the grit to commit to running 3.1 miles, or 6.2 miles, or 26.2 miles that day and see it through. (Also, occasionally, they are cheering for you because their house is on the race route and they've been drinking mimosas or bloody Marys all morning.)

Question 1: Do you run?
If you can answer yes to all these questions,
you are without doubt a real runner.

—ALISTAIR JONES, *Run: A Book for Real Runners*

As Fred Lebow, the founder of the New York City Marathon, said, "In running, it doesn't matter whether you come in first, in the middle of the pack, or last. You can say, 'I have finished.' There is a lot of satisfaction in that." And part of that satisfaction, for some, might be in receiving the finisher's medal many races give out at the end. Yes, everyone gets a finisher's medal, but does that mean the medal is basically just a participation trophy? No, ahem. Hell no, it is not. It took me a lot more effort to get the easiest race finisher's medal I ever earned than it took me to get a participation ribbon in a ninth-grade basketball tournament in which my butt never left the bench. I'm just saying, they're not exactly the same.

Now, there is nothing wrong with a little healthy competition, if that motivates you to do your best and you're not a jerk to other people or yourself. In a race, many people will use another runner as a sort of rabbit to chase, especially in the final miles—meaning, they pick out a runner a few hundred feet ahead, say the one in the orange shirt, and set a goal to try to pass that runner in the next half-mile in order to push themselves when their energy or motivation is flagging. That's a perfectly acceptable thing to do if it helps you reach your goals as a runner. Running laps around the park near your home and bursting into a dead sprint every time someone going slightly faster attempts to pass you, though—that's a little less socially acceptable, maybe even a bit sociopathic.

> *One of the greatest joys of running is how unexpected body shapes manage to run at speeds and distances that seem to bear no relation to their size.*
>
> **—ALEXANDRA HEMINSLEY,**
> *Running Like a Girl: Notes on Learning to Run*

Competing against yourself is actually quite simple. The person you want to be would go for a run instead of sitting inside scrolling through their phone for another forty-five minutes. The person you want to be would not stop halfway through their run because they're tired. The person you want to be would try hard and wouldn't make excuses when things get tough.

Whether you're running 2 miles around your neighborhood or your first 10K, the only person you have to beat is the voice in your head that tells you you're not a runner.

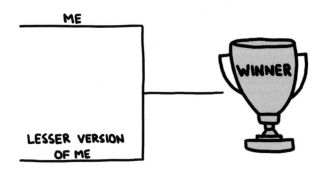

5. GET COMFORT BEING

LE

UNCOMFORTABLE

Avoiding discomfort is the world's worst strategy because it requires choosing discomfort. For example, if you choose to avoid situations that make you anxious, you are choosing anxiety, and strengthening anxiety's ability to control you. If you choose to avoid opportunities that trigger self-doubt, you are choosing self-doubt and convincing self-doubt it is right. . . . Do you want to feel anxiety while avoiding things that have meaning, or do you want to feel anxiety while you do them?

—KELLY McGONIGAL, *"How to Make Stress Your Friend,"* TED Talk, June 2013

L et's be honest: All exercise is uncomfortable in some way. Sure, there are a number of comfortable exercises, like casual walking, and there are plenty of uncomfortable exercises, like hot yoga, but none of them is quite as comfortable as, say, lying in a recliner while eating a bowl of ice cream. Alas, most of us feel the need to exercise, so we pick one form of exercise that kind of makes sense to us and trick ourselves into thinking we like it, whether it's something ridiculous like flipping tractor tires on the sidewalk in front of a CrossFit gym or something ridiculous like running for miles and miles just to end up right where we started.

Either you think doing hard things is worth it to some extent, or you don't. I happen to be in the former category myself, and I'm guessing you are at least somewhat leaning that way too if you've gotten this far in this book—or you're mistaken, and you thought this was a book about actually hating running, and one of these chapters would detail some more comfortable alternative activities, like naps or foot massages.

(To be clear, the pain and discomfort we're talking about here is noninjury pain—the regular, "this is no fun" sort of fatigue you feel and that makes you want to stop running while you're doing it. Not the sharp, "something is wrong" pain you feel when you have an injury. If you're experiencing injury pain, visit a doctor, or consult medical websites until you achieve a state of panic and dread that forces you to visit a doctor.)

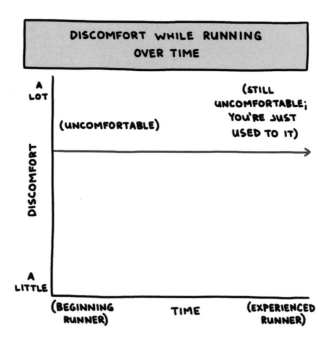

I would never lie to anyone: Running can suck. It can be really painful when you first start doing it, but with enough practice, it's more uncomfortable than painful and you can just run longer before it hurts, or it hurts less because you're more used to it. But, eventually, you start thinking it's kind of fun, or at least meaningful, and the pain becomes worth it. You feel stronger, it feels easier, maybe you even start looking forward to doing it.

That's the key here—to find meaning to the effort and make sure it's worth it for you. Because if the discomfort of running isn't worth it to you, it's basically the same as hitting yourself in the legs with a broomstick. And why would you do that when you just don't have to?

Running, especially outside, will not be fun in lots of ways. It's hard to get out the door when it's too hot or too cold, too snowy, too windy, or really, anything other than just the right conditions. But if you wait for the weather to be "just right" for running, you probably won't run much.

There's an old saying: There's no bad weather, only bad clothing.

You can't change the conditions. All you can change is your clothing and attitude. And I'm not saying that you should have a great attitude about running when the wind chill is 15 degrees or when it's 90 degrees and humid, or that you should have a smile on your face every step. I'm

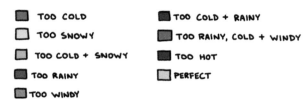

just saying you have to get out the door and get started. You don't have to like it the whole time, or even pretend to enjoy it—although once you get a few minutes into it, you hopefully realize it's not so bad.

There are plenty of products available for dealing with running in harsh weather, and they help. But the most effective tactic is to just get out there, deal with it, and learn. The only proven way to acclimate to cold temperatures is to spend time in cold temperatures. So if it's cold, figure out a layering system that keeps you just warm enough but not sweating. If it's hot, run slower or early in the morning. If it's raining, well, sometimes you just have to get wet. And if there's an active volcano spewing ash and lava over everything in the immediate vicinity, evacuate.

Here's another time-tested saying about long-distance running: You run the first half with your legs, and you run the second half with your head.

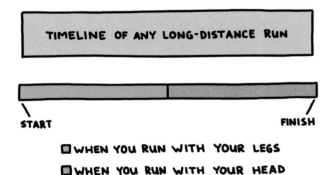

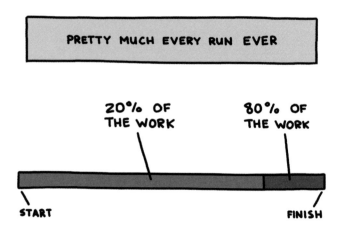

When you're running any distance (not just an ultra-marathon), your morale will go up and down. I think a lot about the 80/20 rule when I'm running. The 80/20 is a maxim about work: The first 80 percent of anything is actually 20 percent of the work, and the last 20 percent is 80 percent of the work.

That last 20 percent can feel way longer than the first 80 percent did, and it can make you feel like quitting way more as well. On many runs, it can be the worst part too. But if you figure out how to get through it every time without quitting, you'll probably find it's the most important part.

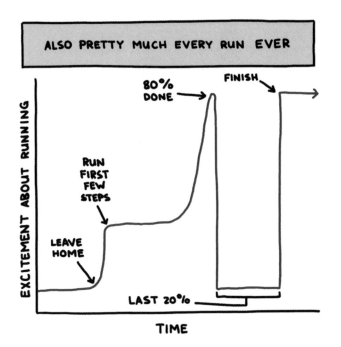

*A lot of time when it's getting harder,
I will just become focused on moving and
reminding myself that I'm fine.
I guess if I had a mantra it might just be
"You're fine, you're fine, you're doing fine,
this is fine."*

—**COURTNEY DAUWALTER, champion ultrarunner**

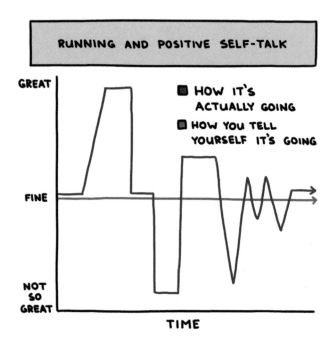

RUNNING AND POSITIVE SELF-TALK

GREAT

■ HOW IT'S
ACTUALLY GOING

■ HOW YOU TELL
YOURSELF IT'S GOING

FINE

NOT
SO
GREAT

TIME

What do you get out of all this time being uncomfortable? Well, a so-called runner's high, for one thing—that feeling of euphoria we get during or after running, which comes from endorphins and other chemicals our bodies produce. That's one nice immediate effect.

But over the long term, after you put yourself through a good amount of discomfort for a few minutes or hours at a time, a couple times a week, something else happens: You build a higher tolerance for pain and challenges in other aspects of your life.

I like to think of it as the "If I Can Run X Miles, Then Y Doesn't Seem So Bad" effect. This effect turns down the volume on other irritants. Maybe standing out in the cold waiting for the bus doesn't seem as bad. Maybe taking the stairs when the escalator is broken doesn't make you feel like you're going to die. Maybe those regular aches and pains you have don't bother you as much, or maybe you don't feel them at all. Maybe public speaking doesn't scare you anymore, or you stop dreading that long weekly work meeting. In short, you get tougher. Not Charlize-Theron-in-*Atomic-Blonde*-tough, like you can disarm and neutralize a dozen would-be assassins in hand-to-hand combat, but a type of tough that's more useful on a daily basis to most of us who aren't, you know, spies tracking down double agents. Spending all that time in the proverbial "pain cave" makes the challenges of regular life a little easier because you've upped your tolerance for discomfort (and probably lowered your resting heart rate too).

It also translates to an ability to run farther. When you start out, if you struggle to get through just a mile or two of running without truly feeling like you're going to die, running 5 miles seems hopelessly impossible. But if you keep at it, after a while, a 1- or 2-mile run becomes tolerable.

Eventually, running 3 miles doesn't seem like a death wish. And then maybe 4, and eventually 5 miles. And when you're running 5 miles and feeling okay about it, a 2-mile run might feel easy, or, dare I say . . . fun? This phenomenon does not happen because the distance got shorter; it happens because you got tougher. And when you get tougher, other things seem less tough.

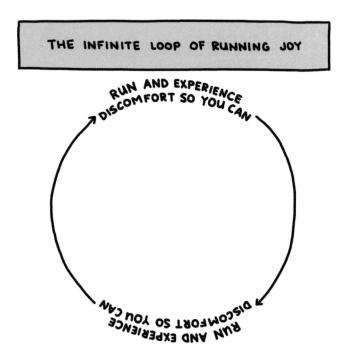

THE INFINITE LOOP OF RUNNING JOY

RUN AND EXPERIENCE DISCOMFORT SO YOU CAN

RUN AND EXPERIENCE DISCOMFORT SO YOU CAN

Pain is inevitable. Suffering is optional.

—HARUKI MURAKAMI,
What I Talk About When I Talk About Running

6. DO THE VERB
YOU

NTIL
BECOME THE NOUN

I could never do that—I'm not a runner.

—Lots of people

Forget the noun, do the verb.

—AUSTIN KLEON,
Keep Going: 10 Ways to Stay Creative in Good Times and Bad

Here's a scenario: You see a job listing and it's a more desirable position than your current job. You've never had a job with this title before, but you meet some, or most, of the qualifications, so you figure you might as well apply for the position. You convince yourself you are qualified for the job.

The company contacts you and invites you in for an interview. Now you have to convince them that you're qualified for the job. They ask something similar to "So, [insert your name here], why would you be a good fit as our next [insert covetable job title here]?" Your response is either:

a. A brief list of things that you think qualify you for the job.

or

b. "Oh, I'm not a [insert covetable job position here]. I could never do that."

Of course the answer is a. You want the job, right? It's a better position, or more money, or a shorter commute, or something—so you do your best to convince yourself and your prospective employer that you're the best candidate for the job. That's what anyone would do.

There's never going to be a job listing for "Runner." You won't have to interview with one or more people who will decide if you're the best candidate. You can't put together a résumé and apply for the role, but if you did, it might look like this:

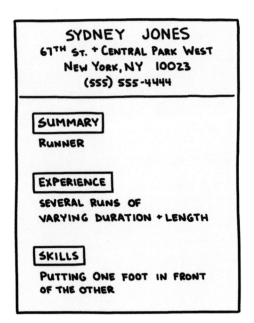

SYDNEY JONES
67TH ST. + CENTRAL PARK WEST
NEW YORK, NY 10023
(555) 555-4444

SUMMARY
RUNNER

EXPERIENCE
SEVERAL RUNS OF
VARYING DURATION + LENGTH

SKILLS
PUTTING ONE FOOT IN FRONT
OF THE OTHER

The only thing you have to do to be a runner is run. That's right. You just do it, and eventually you'll decide you're not just running anymore—you're a runner. Like this:

RUNNING

RUNNING

RUNNING

RUNNING

RUNNING

RUNNING

RUNNING

RUNNING

RUNNING

RUNNING

RUNNING

RUNNING

RUNNING

+ RUNNING
_____

A RUNNER

If you run, you're a runner. Some of us run slow, some of us run less slowly. Some of us run kind of far, some of us run really far. We're all affected by gravity, wind, heat, and what we ate for breakfast. We're all runners, and we're all just out here, doing the same thing, but each of us does it a little bit differently.

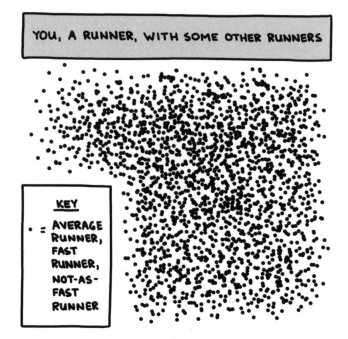

YOU, A RUNNER, WITH SOME OTHER RUNNERS

KEY

. = AVERAGE RUNNER, FAST RUNNER, NOT-AS-FAST RUNNER

I often hear someone say, "I'm not a real runner." We are all runners; some just run faster than others. I have never met a fake runner.

—BART YASSO, former Chief Running Officer,
Runner's World

7. INSPIRATION IS

NOT A STRATEGY

Don't count on motivation.
Count on discipline.

—JOCKO WILLINK, *Discipline Equals Freedom:*
Field Manual

I believe in inspiration, at least as much as the next person who has watched the training montages from the Rocky movies dozens of times. Inspiration is a good thing. It gets us fired up to try something new or different, to start the process of becoming a better person in some way, maybe to set a new goal we're not sure we can accomplish.

What inspiration does not do is get you out of bed to go running when it's dark and cold out. Inspiration also does not stay in our brains at a consistent level once obtained. Sure, you're fired up while you're watching Will Smith deliver one of his monologues in *The Pursuit of Happyness*, pumping your fist, ready to take on the world, but a few days later, that fire hose of inspiration? It's slowed to a trickle. You may have forgotten it altogether. The memory of it is probably not enough to get you through a workout, maybe not even enough to get you to change into your workout clothes. So what do you do?

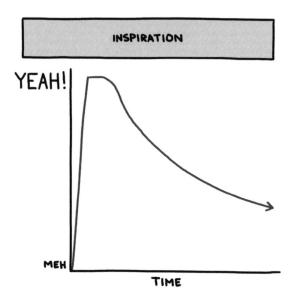

Inspiration is a spark, not a fire. It can light the fire, but you have to keep adding fuel to the fire, every week, to keep it going. Something like this:

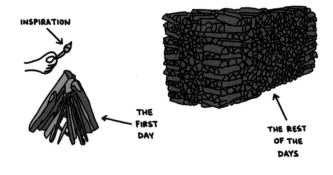

So what keeps you chopping wood to add to the fire—the less-exciting part that doesn't feel as "inspired"?

I recommend a system I learned from my dad, a strategy he developed and used for forty-two years until he retired. It's called showing up for work. He got up at five a.m., six days a week, and did his job. That's it. He just showed up. If you've ever held a job for any length of time, you're probably familiar with this system: You get up and go to work, even on the days you're not, ahem, "inspired" to be there. Some days you really crush it, some days you feel like you never quite get in the groove, but you show up every day.

Running is no different. You show up, you do the work, you get rewarded. Actually, running is a bit different from work, since probably no one's paying you to do it, and there's no free coffee, usually. Running can feel like a grind too, but it provides joy, freedom, clarity, and many other things.

Inspiration is for amateurs. The rest of us just show up and get to work.

—CHUCK CLOSE

I have another tactic that's never let me down, which I call "A Fear-Based Fitness Plan." It's a very simple four-step process:

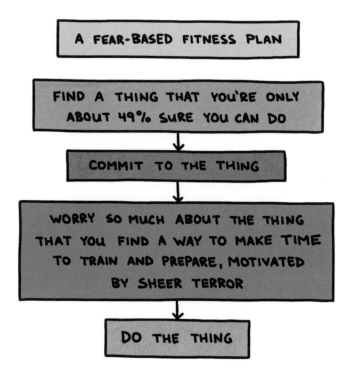

A FEAR-BASED FITNESS PLAN

FIND A THING THAT YOU'RE ONLY ABOUT 49% SURE YOU CAN DO

COMMIT TO THE THING

WORRY SO MUCH ABOUT THE THING THAT YOU FIND A WAY TO MAKE TIME TO TRAIN AND PREPARE, MOTIVATED BY SHEER TERROR

DO THE THING

With this plan, the month leading up to the big thing might look like this:

A FEAR-BASED FITNESS PLAN						
					1 OH SHIT	2 OH SHIT
3 OH SHIT	4 OH SHIT	5 OH SHIT	6 OH SHIT	7 OH SHIT	8 OH SHIT	9 OH SHIT
10 OH SHIT	11 OH SHIT	12 OH SHIT	13 OH SHIT	14 OH SHIT	15 OH SHIT	16 OH SHIT
17 OH SHIT	18 OH SHIT	19 OH SHIT	20 OH SHIT	21 OH SHIT	22 OH SHIT	23 OH SHIT
24 OH SHIT	25 OH SHIT	26 OH SHIT	27 OH SHIT	28 OH SHIT	29 OH SHIT	30 BIG SCARY THING
31						

The big scary thing on your calendar should in no way be keeping you up at night, giving you heart palpitations, panic attacks, or anxiety (we're trying to become better people, not ruin our lives). But it should be scary. Ambitious. Enough to motivate you to prepare for it, enough to make you get out and do the work instead of making excuses. Because when the day of the big thing comes, all the excuses you can think of don't matter—only the math of whether you are prepared or not matters.

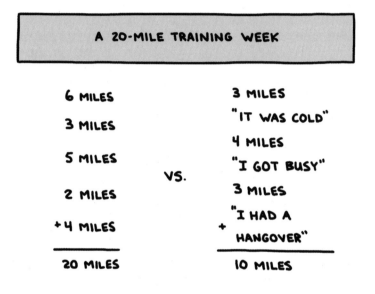

A 20-MILE TRAINING WEEK

6 MILES

3 MILES

5 MILES

2 MILES

+ 4 MILES
_____

20 MILES

VS.

3 MILES

"IT WAS COLD"

4 MILES

"I GOT BUSY"

3 MILES

"I HAD A HANGOVER"
_____

10 MILES

We all have someone in our lives we never want to let down. Maybe it's our kids, or our boss, or our spouse, or perhaps all of them. Whoever it is, we always find a way to show up for them, as promised—on time, no flaking, no excuses.

When it comes to running, you have to become the person you don't want to let down. You get a few minutes or an hour a few times a week when you put yourself first, and you don't flake. You show up for yourself.

If your goal is to run 4 miles on Tuesday, you run those 4 miles on Tuesday. You don't skip it, the same as you wouldn't leave your kids standing outside school wondering where you are when you told them you'd pick them up. "Accountability" isn't nearly as dreamy of a word as "inspiration," but I'd argue it's far more important.

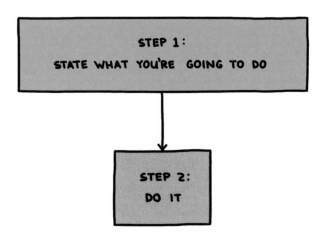

ACCOUNTABILITY
A FLOW CHART

STEP 1:
STATE WHAT YOU'RE GOING TO DO

STEP 2:
DO IT

8. WRITE YOUR OV

DEFINITION OF SUCCESS

It's very hard in the beginning to understand that the whole idea is not to beat the other runners. Eventually you learn that the competition is against the little voice inside you that wants you to quit.

—DR. GEORGE SHEEHAN, author and columnist for *Runner's World*

Here's an old sports saying you might have heard before: "Second place is the first loser."

It's a saying that is supposed to motivate you to win, but it also reduces the many reasons for playing to one: winning. Like many people, I played sports while growing up, and also like many people, none of the teams I was on ever won a championship. Not in any sport. Did I get something out of all those hours of physical activity? I like to think so. Learning teamwork, for example, and having fun with my friends, even though we were technically "losers."

In the Western States 100, the world's first and arguably most famous 100-mile trail-running race, runners have thirty hours to finish the course. Every year, the winners finish sometime between fourteen and twenty hours. The three-hundred-plus other entrants finish sometime in the ten-hour range after that, and around fifty people don't finish at all. A few runners make it across the finish line in what's called the "Golden Hour," the hour between 29:00:00 and the final cutoff at 30:00:00.

In 2015, a seventy-year-old runner named Gunhild Swanson had one of the most dramatic finishes ever. As she entered the Placer High School track for the final quarter mile of the 100.2-mile race, she had a dozen people running with her, and the hundreds of spectators waiting in the stadium erupted in cheers. People lining the track glanced back and forth from the official race clock to Swanson as she cranked around the oval, and dozens of people ran across the infield to the finish line, screaming, cheering, and holding cameras and phones high to try to capture the moment.

Swanson ran under the finish arch at 29:59:54, with only six seconds remaining. The crowd exploded in cheers; people hugged one another, raised their fists in the air, and screamed and clapped, in a scene you might expect after a ninth-inning two-out home run to win the World Series in Game 7. Except Gunhild Swanson had just taken last place in the race. The overall winner of the race, Rob Krar, had finished more than fifteen hours earlier, but even he got swept up in the moment and ran part of the final mile with Swanson too.

If you were standing in the crowd that day or have ever watched internet videos of Gunhild Swanson's "Golden

Minute," I don't think there's any way you'd think she's a "loser." In fact, I'd argue that she was the 254th winner of the 2015 Western States 100.

Here's a neat thing about running as an adult: Most of us have almost zero chance at winning a race, so we have to figure out another reason to run, or a way to be "successful" at it besides taking home a first-place medal.

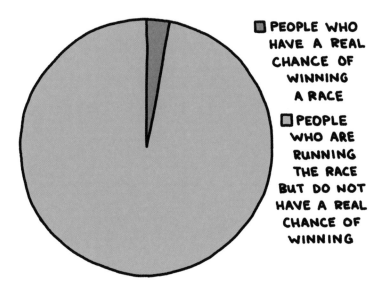

☐ PEOPLE WHO HAVE A REAL CHANCE OF WINNING A RACE

☐ PEOPLE WHO ARE RUNNING THE RACE BUT DO NOT HAVE A REAL CHANCE OF WINNING

Here's another chart:

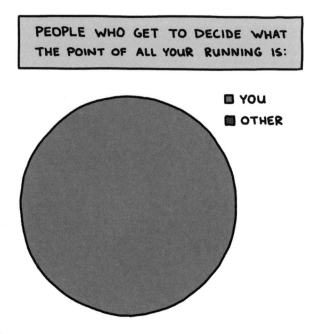

PEOPLE WHO GET TO DECIDE WHAT THE POINT OF ALL YOUR RUNNING IS:

☐ YOU
☐ OTHER

If you enter a road race, spectators will probably give you no choice about receiving encouragement or not—they will very likely cheer for you, a complete stranger. In fact, if you'd like to have someone cheer for you during an athletic endeavor as an adult, I recommend running a race. If you write your name on your bib or shirt, people will even cheer for you by name. They do not care if you're in 3rd place or 3,000th place—they're psyched for you to just be out there.

Of course, you don't have to enter a race to succeed at running. Ever. You can run 3 miles one day a week or 130 miles a week and take only one day off. You can push yourself to get faster, or you can relax and just enjoy being outside and moving. Hell, you can run backward the entire time if you want to. Setting a goal, sticking to it, and achieving it, whatever it is, equals success.

Running gives you freedom. You don't have to report to your boss about how it's going, you don't get graded on your performance or results, you don't have to tell anyone about it, and you don't have to share anything about it on social media (but you can, if you want to). You get to decide how hard you want to push yourself and what running means to you.

Running is different for everyone. If you've signed up for a turkey trot and your three-year-old child asks what you are going to do in the event, you would not pull up a video of Gail Devers winning the 100-meter race at the 1996 Summer Olympics and say, "See that? That's running. That's what I'm going to do today." You might, though, remind your child of the running thing they've seen you doing, and say you're going to do that but with a whole bunch of other people.

Running means something unique to each of us. It's not a concrete objective thing like, for example, a 2005 Honda Civic Sedan.

MY 2005 HONDA CIVIC SEDAN	BOSTON MARATHON QUALIFIER'S 2005 HONDA CIVIC SEDAN
• PRETTY GOOD GAS MILEAGE	• PRETTY GOOD GAS MILEAGE
• COMPACT	• COMPACT
• RELIABLE	• RELIABLE
• 4-CYLINDER ENGINE	• 4-CYLINDER ENGINE
• 4 DOORS	• 4 DOORS
• 4 WHEELS	• 4 WHEELS
• 4 TIRES	• 4 TIRES
• 2 HEADLIGHTS	• 2 HEADLIGHTS
• SEAT BELTS	• SEAT BELTS

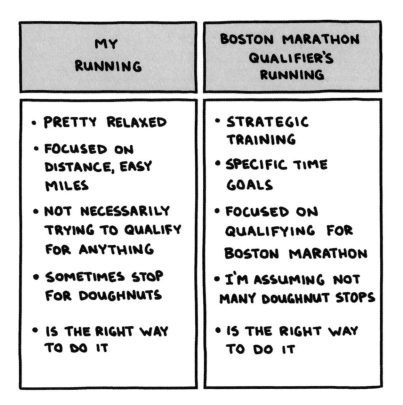

There's no correct way to be successful as a runner. One year you can be a runner with no specific goals, and in the next year you can be a runner who is motivated to qualify for a marathon.

Alex Lowe, one of the most accomplished mountain climbers of all time, once famously said, "The best climber in the world is the one who's having the most fun." I think that ethos can apply to anything we do, including running.

Getting faster and/or performing at your physical limit are only a couple of reasons people run. If you are holding on to old, negative, or painful memories of feeling pressure to run fast (Presidential physical fitness test, gym class, track practice, and so on), let me tell you, no one cares if you run fast but you. The trick is to find a way to be the runner having the most fun. There's nothing wrong with trying to run as fast as you can, but there's also nothing wrong with creating your own definition of success. You can, for example, decide that for you success means:

- Running three times a week for a month, or for a year
- Running a certain total distance per week
- Training so you can finish a 10K without stopping
- Showing up for a local group run and meeting new friends
- Running a certain number of minutes per week without worrying about distance

- Running and walking outside a certain number of minutes per week but not worrying about how much you're running or how much you're walking

- Being able to run to the top of a particular hill without stopping

- Running enough to accomplish the goals set on the running app you use

- Running enough to wear out a pair of running shoes

- Sticking to a schedule for six weeks, 100 percent attendance, no excuses

- Being able to move a few miles under your own power and being grateful for that

Winning is great—I mean, not that I would know. That's just what I've heard people say. But millions of people are runners, and only a tiny fraction of us technically win. The rest of us keep running, though, so there must be some other reason to do it, right? That reason is whatever you decide it is.

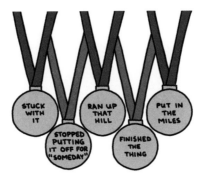

9. PROGRESS IS

NOT A
STRAIGHT LINE

Fall seven times and stand up eight.

—Japanese proverb

*Knock me down nine times
but I get up ten, bitch.*

—CARDI B

You've probably heard this before from someone way smarter than me: Things don't always work out the way you plan them. When you initially dream up something, the vision in your head is clear: Start at point A, follow steps, finish at point B. But does it ever work out that cleanly? Most people would tell you that even the most meticulously planned life doesn't happen without surprises or detours or in the order they imagined—both good and bad. On a smaller-scale personal level, I somehow can't seem to get through the most straightforward new dinner recipe without surprises or detours or in the order I imagined (and no recipe ever says anything about pausing to turn off the smoke alarm, for some reason). Same goes for a trip to the DMV, or a complicated travel itinerary, or a training plan for a running goal.

We envision a plan like this:

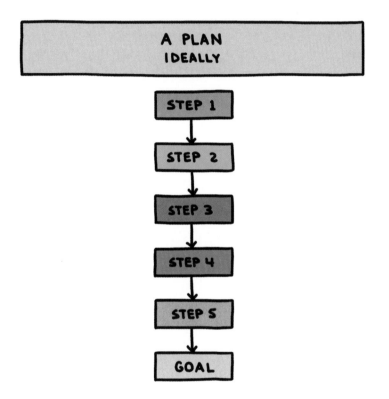

But by the end, after all the hiccups and adjustments, it looks more like this:

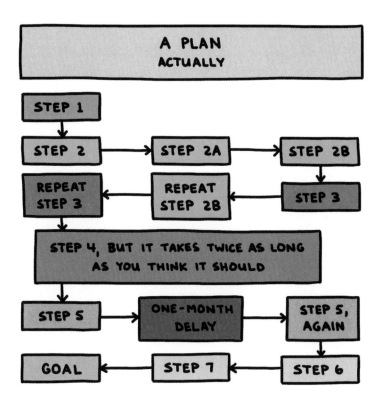

Our ideas about running are no different. Sometimes, just when we're really hitting our stride and feeling on top of the world, we look down to see that our shoe has come untied. Our short after-work run is abruptly interrupted by a gastrointestinal emergency. We get shin splints or develop plantar fasciitis halfway through the training plan for our first big race goal.

We all have different specific reasons for running, but none of us is doing it to get worse. We all want to improve in some way, whether it's running faster or farther, or just making our week a little better by jogging for a few miles to clear our head.

When I do have a goal in mind, my idea of progress looks like this:

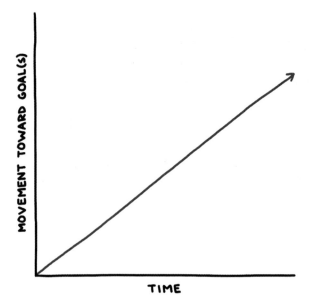

I don't know about you, but no notable goal I have ever reached has ever had a process that direct, clean, and smooth. It always has a few sticking points, setbacks small and not so small. I see two different ways to deal with a setback. One is giving up:

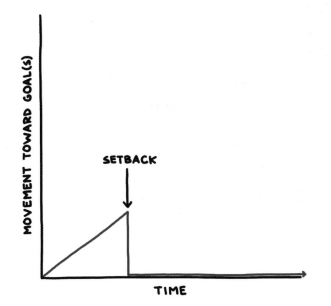

Of course, if you throw your hands up and quit every time you face a minor or major setback, life is going to be pretty rough and potentially very unrewarding. Your other option is to view the setback as a pause button on your way to your goal.

That looks more like this:

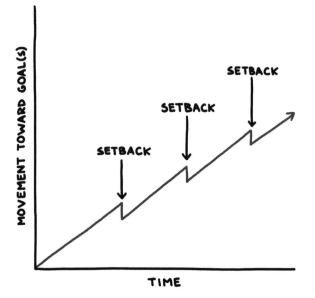

Injuries aren't fun. Getting sick the week before your big race isn't fun. No one is excited to postpone a big goal or race to the next year because of shin splints or a shake-up at work. Recalibrating our dreams is frustrating at first, and it's usually not rewarding until we look back on it and are able to tell ourselves it presented another opportunity, or ended up being the right thing to happen after all, or taught us something we wouldn't have otherwise learned.

For most of us, ideally, running is a long-term pursuit. If it is, having to adjust our expectations and move something to next year, or to next month, or to a different race, will be a speed bump. If it's a big speed bump, abruptly jarring our trajectory for the year of running we had planned, it can feel like this:

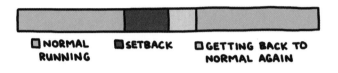

□ NORMAL
RUNNING

■ SETBACK

□ GETTING BACK TO
NORMAL AGAIN

That's a big chunk of your year to be interrupted, and definitely a huge bummer. But if you keep running for five years, here's what that big setback looks like:

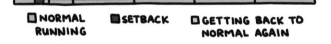

□ NORMAL
RUNNING

■ SETBACK

□ GETTING BACK TO
NORMAL AGAIN

The setback is much less of a big deal in that span of time, if you're playing the long game. By the time you get to the fifth year, you may have trouble remembering when exactly that big setback happened, and you might hear yourself saying, "Four or five years ago I had an injury . . . "

Now, if you can go five years and have only one setback that keeps you from running, well, that's pretty lucky. If you have more than that, don't fret (or quit). It's not because "you're not cut out for running" or something—it's just normal. Running, like anything else worth doing, is a learning process, and you're learning while doing it. In the case of an injury or other setback, you're also learning while not doing it: what to do differently next time to prevent the injury from recurring, how to stay in shape to smooth your re-entry when you can run again, or, perhaps, just how much you miss running. Which makes our progress chart look more like this:

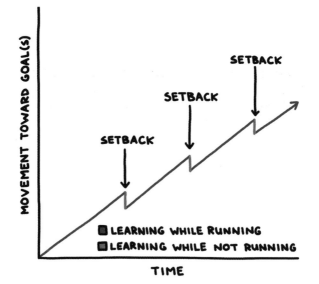

An injury can make it feel like you're not sticking with running, especially in the short term. When the weather is nice and you feel trapped indoors, you might feel as if you're missing out. But giving an injury time to heal properly, or being patient in the face of a hiccup that life throws at you and puts your running on hold, is how you develop the resilience to stay in the game for the long term. One bad year is a huge bummer if you only run for one year—but if you run for many years, one bad year isn't the end of the world.

10. IT'S ONLY HA

LF ABOUT RUNNING

Running has taught me that the pursuit of a passion matters more than the passion itself. Immerse yourself in something deeply and with heartfelt intensity—continually improve, never give up—this is fulfillment, this is success.

—DEAN KARNAZES, *Ultramarathon Man: Confessions of an All-Night Runner*

Running a race requires a lot of what I call "invisible work"—miles and miles and hours and hours of running before you even get to the starting line. When people say, "Wow, you did a hundred-mile ultramarathon? That's a lot of running." I joke, "No shit. I had to run twelve hundred miles before I even got to the starting line."

Which is, I think, probably how everyone who has run a race feels. Preparing to run a long distance on a certain day in the future requires a lot more preparation than, say, preparing to go to an amusement park—unless you're not tall enough this summer to be allowed to ride the Millennium 3000 Adrenal Blaster roller coaster, in which case you'll have a year of anticipation (and hopefully a growth spurt). Running long distances just takes more preparation time.

It's almost comical how much training you have to do in order to run an irrational distance. Think about a typical half-marathon training plan, in which you train for twelve weeks leading up to race day.

This block represents the half-marathon distance you're planning to run:

13.1

Over the span of a typical twelve-week training plan, you'll cover about 175 miles. If we break down those 175 miles into similar-sized blocks, the whole twelve weeks of training looks like this:

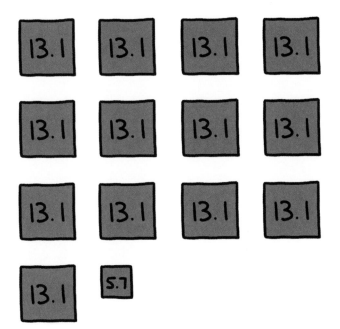

Look at all that training mileage compared to the actual mileage of your race.

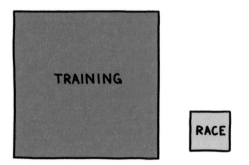

Let's say, just for a nice round number, that you run ten-minute miles during all your training runs and your race. You would spend a total of 29:20 hours just running your training miles, and 2:11 hours running your race at the end of all that.

That looks like a lot of practice for one little thing at the end, doesn't it? Sure it does. But think about it like this: If you were tasked with giving a twenty-minute presentation at your job, would you think it was ridiculous to spend four and a half hours working on it before you delivered it in front of everyone? Probably not.

The ratio of training to miles isn't the point here, though. If you sign up for a race, you'll probably spend a lot of time focusing on the actual race day—thinking about whether you'll finish, what it will feel like, what you should wear, what new aches and pains will pop up, how you'll mentally and physically deal with running farther than you ever have before.

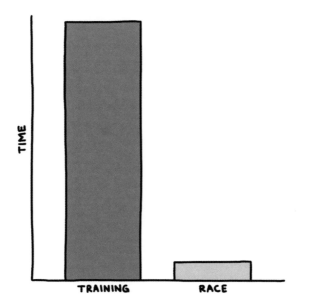

But.

The race is not the point of all this training. The running is. You spend dozens of hours running around your neighborhood or local trails with the goal of preparing for a race. You push yourself and improve all that time—even if some days you feel like garbage and it feels like a chore and your heart isn't in it (and your body barely is).

Running is great if your goal is to get in shape or help burn off the nachos you ate yesterday. But it's even better when it's about something bigger or more meaningful. Maybe you use it to develop mental toughness that will carry over into the rest of your life. Maybe you want to prove someone wrong (or right). Maybe you want to set an example for your kids. Maybe you want to prove it to yourself that you can do it. Maybe you want to take on something big and scary with a friend and keep each other accountable to train for it. Maybe you've never experienced chafing until you bleed, and you're curious about what that feels like . . . or maybe not. Whatever reason you have, the point is: The race is not the point. The process of getting there is.

We've traditionally thought that the reward of working is what comes at the end of all the hard work—like this:

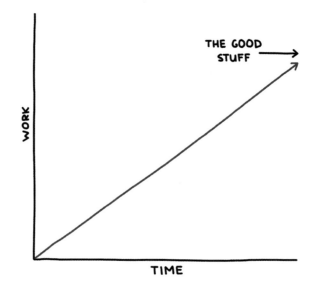

And sure, that's true. But if you pay attention, some of the reward is during the process—like this:

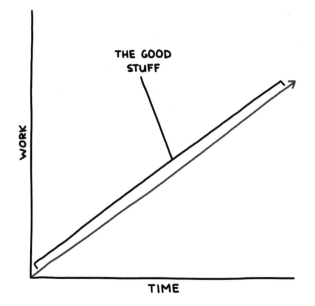

If you stick with it, you will likely have some negative side effects like stiff joints and muscles, some calluses, a new hatred for the alarm clock that wakes you up for your training runs. But you will have many more positive side effects, most of which you may not have imagined at the start of your training. You might notice you're sleeping better at night, or that you feel less stressed, or that you have more patience, or that food tastes a little better after having run, or that you actually like the aches and pains you have the day after a long run because they tell you that you worked hard.

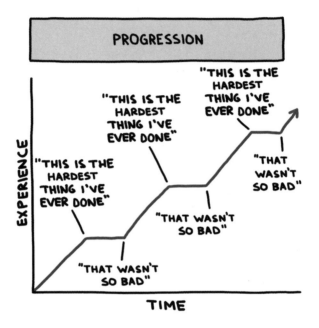

Whatever the distance of your race, you'll most likely get a T-shirt or a medal or a belt buckle. Whatever it is, you probably won't wear it every day. What you will wear every day, or at least have with you every day, are the things you have learned during the process, the small ways you've improved physically and mentally, and probably a little bit more confidence.

Once you have taught yourself that running isn't about breaking boundaries that you thought you could never smash, and realized that it is about discovering those boundaries were never there in the first place, you can apply it to anything.

—ALEXANDRA HEMINSLEY, *Running Like a Girl: Notes on Learning to Run*

In a 2017 interview on the podcast *WTF with Marc Maron*, Bruce Springsteen spoke about learning to make music in his twenties and thirties as a "project of self-realization" in which he could measure his personal progress through music. For Springsteen, making music is a process of "Is it getting better, am I getting better, am I becoming more realized as a musician and, therefore, hopefully as a human being?"

Springsteen's retrospection can be applied to running as well. Anyone who starts running and sticks with it for a few months or years will improve in other ways while improving as a runner: You begin to understand

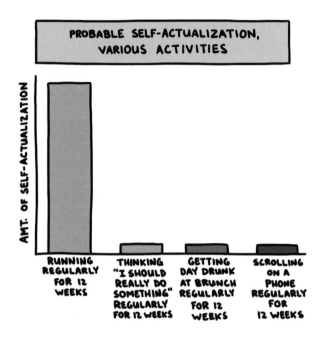

commitment, you develop patience, and maybe you even learn a little bit of self-discipline. Even if all you get out of it is proof that you can stick with something difficult and see it through, that's something.

Sure, part of the process is about the miles, proper hydration, the finish line, and maybe keeping tabs on how fast you go and how fast you get, but if you don't become a better, more realized person while doing it—well, then, you're missing something.

Most of us have enough areas in our lives where we have to meet others' expectations. Let your running be about your own hopes and dreams.

—MEB KEFLEZIGHI, Olympic medalist and New York City Marathon winner, *Meb for Mortals: How to Run, Think, and Eat Like a Champion Marathoner*

11. THEF

ARE NO "HACKS"

*You know, I actually never trained at all—
I just bought these high-tech shoes and drank
this new sports drink, and somehow
I ended up winning the race.*

—No one, ever

As sports go, running is pretty fair. It takes a lot of work, the way that learning a new language or how to play the guitar is a lot of work. The equation, something you may have seen on the wall of a gym, looks like this:

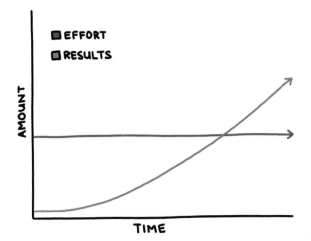

PUTTING IN THE WORK

■ EFFORT
■ RESULTS

AMOUNT

TIME

With running, if you put in effort over time, you generally get results. Sure, there are fast people and there are less-fast people, but everyone is working for it. For example, think about elite marathoners. They're not coasting on their natural talent to win races; they're running 80- to 100-mile training weeks. Compare that to a typical "beginner" marathon training plan, which usually maxes out at 40 miles per week (and that is still a hell of a lot of miles!).

There are training plans for every race distance—some have high running mileage, some have low running mileage, but none of them has no running mileage. Becoming a runner isn't like becoming a member of an airline's loyalty program. You can't just sit around for months eating chips and watching Netflix and then one day spend ninety seconds filling out an online form and, voilà, you're in. Running takes ambition and attendance. You do it regularly so you can keep doing it regularly.

We've gotten used to buying things that will help us do any task better, faster, and easier, from peeling garlic and mowing the lawn to cleaning our house and, especially, almost all forms of exercising. Whether we find these products through a late-night infomercial or a clickbait web ad, the promise they try to sell you looks something like this:

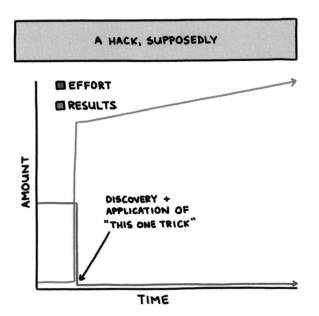

A HACK, SUPPOSEDLY

☐ EFFORT
☐ RESULTS

AMOUNT

DISCOVERY +
APPLICATION OF
"THIS ONE TRICK"

TIME

Running is no different. Lots of companies would be happy to sell you things that might help you run: shoes, apparel, water bottles, Bluetooth earbuds, massagers, foam rollers, and space-age foods and drink mixes. But we haven't figured out a way to pay someone else to run all the training miles while we get all the benefits without putting in any of those miles ourselves. You can't take the effort out of the equation. And the more you run, the more you'll realize that putting in the effort actually is one of the benefits.

THE ZEN OF RUNNING

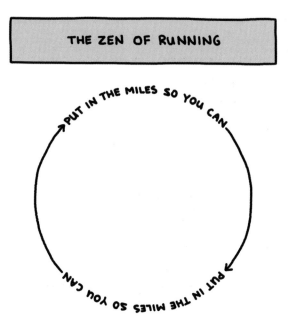

PUT IN THE MILES SO YOU CAN PUT IN THE MILES SO YOU CAN

When I feel far too busy or overwhelmed with life to possibly consider going for a run, I go anyway, and I know two things will always happen:

1. Five or ten minutes into the run, the feeling of being overwhelmed and too busy will be gone.

2. I have more hope for the world fifteen minutes after I finish running than I did five minutes before I started. If that's all I get out of a run, that's still pretty good.

Running is the greatest metaphor for life,
because you get out of it what you put into it.

—OPRAH WINFREY

12. F#%K BUSY

*If you want something done,
ask a busy person to do it.*

—Unknown

QUESTION 1: Are you busy?

Me too. Everyone seems to be nowadays.

QUESTION 2: Are you too busy to find time to run?

If you answered yes, you're too busy to run consistently, either:

a. That's true and you really need to find some balance in your life.

or

b. You're lying. A little bit or a lot.

Look, you're not just lying to me; you're lying to yourself. You feel as if you don't have time, but you're probably not trying very hard to make time, either. So could you *make* time, or are you just too busy?

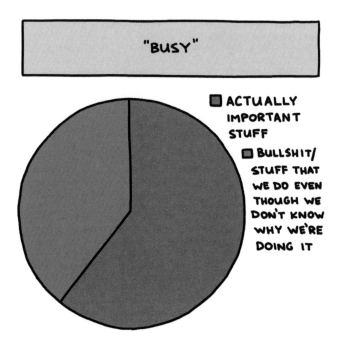

"BUSY"

☐ ACTUALLY IMPORTANT STUFF

☐ BULLSHIT/ STUFF THAT WE DO EVEN THOUGH WE DON'T KNOW WHY WE'RE DOING IT

Nobody ever says, "I just need to find more time to dedicate to the apps on my phone." But we spend (depending on which study you read) somewhere between ninety minutes and five hours on our phones per day. Where does all that time come from?

Do you ever pull out your phone to check something and then realize that forty-five minutes have passed by? Yeah, me neither. Okay, yes, I do that. I steal time from myself, unintentionally, in small increments. Am I busy? I mean, I feel busy a lot of the time. Am I efficient with my time? Well, sometimes. Could I be better about it? Absolutely.

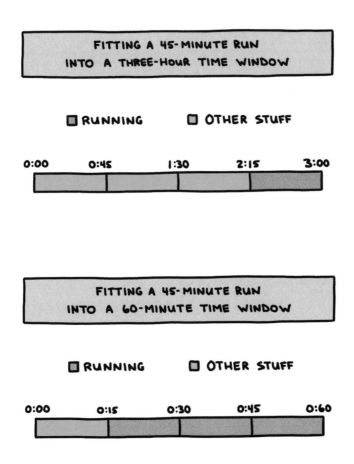

If you think you're busy, look around. I'm guessing you'll find someone who has less time than you and is doing more with it.

Take Liza Howard, for example. Howard is a running coach, a mother of two elementary-school-age kids, and a professional ultrarunner. She has managed to squeeze in enough training—on treadmills, on a short loop in her neighborhood, wherever she can, whenever she can—to win multiple 100-mile races over the years. "It's like a snowball that builds as it rolls down a hill," she says. "Every little bit counts."

Your goals don't always have to be big, though. Our lives change, things happen, and not every year is the best year to do it all and set running goals that require a lot of time. If you have way too much going on, maybe it's your year to dial things back and do only enough consistent running to keep your baseline fitness, or perhaps it's the year that you start from zero and gradually figure out how to work a small, consistent amount of running into your schedule.

No matter what your goal is, if you make running a priority, you will find time to run. If you want to do it badly enough, you will steal the time to do it, in whatever increments possible within your schedule. You can look at your idea of being busy, give busy the middle finger, and get out there.

One of these days is none of these days.

—Unknown

13. LOVING SOM
DIFFER

HING IS
IT THAN LIKING IT

*Riding my bike in the rain is like a
bad relationship. I don't like it, but I love it.*

—JASON "WOODY" WOOD

When I do speaking engagements about the parallels between work and ultrarunning, I often ask the audience to raise their hands if they have children.

"Okay," I say, "keep your hand in the air if you love your kids."

Everyone's hand stays up.

"Okay, then," I say, "keep your hand in the air if you like your kids a hundred percent of the time."

Almost all the hands go down, and people laugh. I look at the people with their hands still raised and tell them that we all know they are lying.

We've all probably realized that loving someone doesn't necessarily mean you like them all the time—even the most doting parents aren't smitten with their kids every moment of their entire lives. But that's okay—loving someone or something is not the same thing as liking it. You can love your job without liking the Wednesday-afternoon staff meetings or the Friday report you write up and send every week even though you're pretty sure your boss never reads it. You love your kids even though they do things that frustrate you from time to time or occasionally cause permanent and somewhat costly damage to your property. (Right, Mom?)

So love might look like this if you were referring to, say, your kids or your favorite baseball team or even your job:

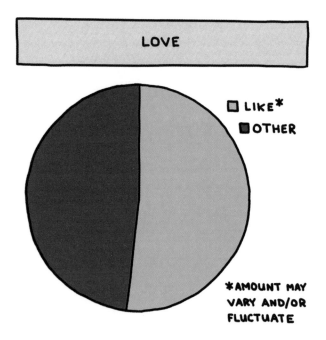

If my personal experience proves anything, it's that we can love running without liking it some of the time. Actually, most of the time. I like having run. I am not sure if I like running. For the first fifty minutes of a run, I'm pretty sure I don't like it at all. Something flips after about fifty minutes and I actually enjoy it for a little while. So my pie chart for "loving" running probably looks more like this:

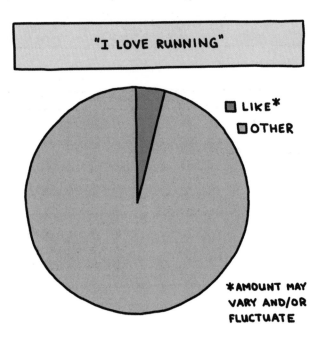

Sure, I have a little fun after I've been running for a while. But getting started? I am usually as excited about going for a run as I am about flossing my teeth. This might be why it takes me forever to get out the door and run those first few steps, even after I've been dressed and ready to go for a half hour (okay, an hour sometimes).

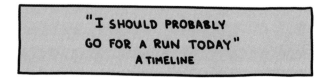

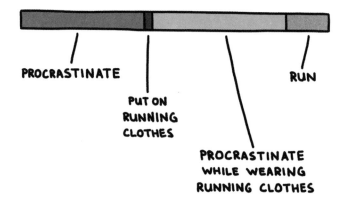

Falling in love with running is much different than falling in love with a person. In fact, I'd say there really isn't any part that resembles the "falling" you might have felt the first time you see a beautiful stranger across a room, or during a moment on a third date when you realized you might want to go on a thousand more dates with that person.

Picking up running is less falling in love and more, say, slogging into love. You start, it sucks, you feel good after you're done, you repeat that process several times, and then it's not so bad. You keep doing it through the not-so-bad phase, and then you actually start to like it a little bit. One day, you start to think you can't live without it and, strangely, you might . . . love running?

Love is open to interpretation, which is obvious if you think about the thousands of songs that have been written about it. Running has a lot of similarities to loving another person—you can go head over heels for it, you can start too fast, you can unintentionally neglect it, you can be on-and-off for years, and it can be a constant companion in good times and bad. Running will never, however, lawyer up, take you to court, or one day leave you for a personal trainer who's way too young for it. With running, your love story may not look like anyone else's, and that's okay, because you get to write it yourself, and the story can be whatever you want it to be.

EPILOGUE

THERE IS NO RIGHT WAY TO DO IT

It's easy to get anxious about all the details we've thought up to complicate running: How much should I run? What shoes should I wear? What food should I eat before/ during/after my runs? How fast should I go? Should I follow a training program?

If you spend a few minutes clicking around the internet, you can probably develop a complex about any aspect of your personal running program. While I don't pretend to have answers for what works best for all runners, there are some universal truths that apply to everyone. What I've learned about running I've learned very slowly, through my own trial-and-error process, and that is: Take it mostly easy. Walk when you need to. Eat when you need to, and if something you eat makes you frantically stop to find a restroom in the middle of your run, stop eating it. I am gradually figuring out the difference between normal pain and injuries, and also gradually figuring out how to dress myself and run in cold temperatures and hot temperatures.

I assume every runner is somewhere different in the process, but we're all still figuring things out as we go, even if we've been running for decades.

Try to remember, even if you haven't been running your whole life or since high school, that running *is* part of our DNA. Humans have been running for thousands of years, so at some level, your body knows how to do it. As you go, you will find ways to do it a little bit better. In my opinion, there's no better way to learn than by just trying, which is what I'll be doing. See you out there.

RESOURCES

I'm just a guy who likes to run long distances. I am not a coach, dietitian, or a doctor. These resources can help answer the more technical questions you might have about running, racing, trail running, or ultrarunning.

BOOKS

Born to Run by Christopher McDougall

The Happy Runner: Love the Process, Get Faster, Run Longer by David Roche and Megan Roche, MD

Relentless Forward Progress by Bryon Powell

The Run-Walk-Run Method by Jeff Galloway

The Trail Runner's Companion by Sarah Lavender Smith

The Ultimate Beginner's Running Guide: The Key to Running Inspired by Ryan Robert

PODCASTS

The Morning Shakeout Podcast

The Rambling Runner Podcast

Running for Real Podcast with Tina Muir

Ten Junk Miles

Ultrarunnerpodcast

WEBSITES

IRunFar.com

RunnersWorld.com

TrailRunner.com

TrailSisters.net

Ultrarunning.com

WomensRunning.com

ACKNOWLEDGMENTS

Thank you to Judy Pray, Bella Lemos, Jane Treuhaft, Carson Lombardi, and the rest of the team at Artisan Books for making this book a real thing I can share with other people.

Thanks to all my friends who put in miles with me over the past several years while the ideas in this book were bouncing around my head: Jayson, Forest, Syd, Nick, Brody, Dave, Hilary, and Rowlf.

And thanks to my mom, Kathy, for being the first adult I knew who was a runner, and who let me wear her old Asics running shoes for those brief magical few months when my feet were roughly the same size as hers (in 1991?) so I could feel like a real runner.